END-OF-LIFE CARE
WITH ESSENTIAL OILS
Your Guide to Compassionate Care for
Loved Ones and Their Caregivers

End-of-Life Care with Essentials Oils: Your Guide to Compassionate Care for Loved Ones and Their Caregivers/ Scott A. Johnson

ISBN-13: 978-0997548730

ISBN-10: 0997548738

Cover Design: Scott A. Johnson
Cover Copyright: © Scott A. Johnson 2018

Discover more books by Scott A. Johnson at authorscott.com

Published by Scott A. Johnson Professional Writing Services LLC: Orem, Utah

DISCLAIMERS OF WARRANTY AND LIMITATION OF LIABILITY

The author provides all information on an "as is" and "as available" basis and for informational purposes only. The author makes no representations or warranties of any kind, expressed or implied, as to the information, materials, or products mentioned. Every effort has been made to ensure accuracy and completeness of the information contained; however, it is not intended to replace any medical advice or to halt proper medical treatment, nor diagnose, treat, cure, or prevent any health condition or disease.

Always consult a qualified medical professional before using any dietary supplement or natural product, engaging in physical activity, or modifying your diet; and seek the advice of your physician with any questions you may have regarding any medical condition. Always consult your OB/GYN if you are pregnant or think you may become pregnant before using any dietary supplement or natural product, and to ensure you are healthy enough for exercise or any dietary modifications. The information contained in this book is for educational and informational purposes only, and it is not meant to replace medical advice, diagnosis, or treatment in any manner. Never delay or disregard professional medical advice. Use the information solely at your own risk; the author accepts no responsibility for the use thereof. This book is sold with the understanding that neither the author nor publisher shall be liable for any loss, injury, or harm allegedly arising from any information or suggestion in this book.

The Food and Drug Administration (FDA) has not evaluated the statements contained in this book. The information and materials are not meant to diagnose, prescribe, or treat any disease, condition, illness, or injury.

For the dedicated hospice professionals and caregivers who tirelessly provide compassionate care to those departing mortality.

To my dear wife and children who don't receive the recognition and praise they deserve, nor the credit, for allowing me to share my God-given gifts of writing and natural medicine with the world.

TABLE OF CONTENTS

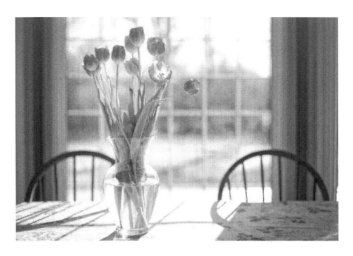

The flood of varying emotions after a loved one is diagnosed with a terminal illness or injury is like a roller-coaster ride. Sorrow, fear, and uncertainty are just a few of the emotions felt when deciding the best approach to care for your loved one in his or her final months, weeks, and hours of life. However, each of us will face this reality at some point in our lives, so we should be sufficiently prepared to navigate this demanding situation.

Part of this preparation involves gaining a deeper understanding of what occurs during the end of life. Knowing this allows you to successfully prepare for the most commonly experienced circumstances. While the focus is your dying loved one, your planning should also include your own personal wellness and care. You can't pour water from an empty pitcher. Without a focus on your own health and well-being, you will be unable to provide the compassionate care you desire to give your loved one.

Only the very wise are able to prepare themselves emotionally far in advance of the death we each experience. Our first brush with death is often shocking and emotionally chaotic. To a certain extent, it is impossible to fully prepare emotionally for the loss of a loved one. Overwhelming emotions can easily overcome you and negatively affect your mental state. Surrounding yourself with a network of caring people is of great support and imperative to end-of-life care.

Spiritually, embracing long-cherished beliefs concerning the continuity of human beings after death diminishes the sting of death. And an unbending faith that you will see your loved one again is comforting and provides a sense of reassurance during the emotional chaos. Indeed, professionals who work with those who are dying frequently report people with deep and abiding faith navigate the dying process with greater poise.

Along with emotional, mental, and spiritual preparation, physical preparation is necessary. We must have tools organized for us to traverse the highs and lows that will inevitably come. One such tool is essential oils. Essential oils are uniquely qualified to provide end-of-life support for your loved one, yourself, and his or her caregivers. As complex multitarget, multimechanism molecules, they have the exceptional ability to influence numerous aspects of well-being: physical, mental, emotional, and spiritual.

Dying is a normal—and necessary—part of life, but it doesn't mean it will be easy for the individual, families, or communities. The substantial impact of death in modern society is largely underestimated. Death can profoundly influence and have a major impact on local families or expand to the entire world depending on the events surrounding the death and the people involved. The death of a loved one may bring together people with strained relationships— perhaps some who haven't spoken in many years. Regrets may be compartmentalized or expressed verbally concerning matters that occurred between the dying individual and family or friends. Truly, most people fail to recognize the full significance of death until they are in the middle of it.

Those facing the end of their lives have complex needs. They deserve respect and compassion and to receive care that emphasizes their dignity, comfort, and quality of life. Care continues despite the discontinuation of active medical testing and disease or injury treatment. It should focus on a range of needs including the social, psychological, physical, and spiritual. Whenever possible, family members and friends should be intimately involved in comfort and support to someone nearing the end of mortal life. This journey toward death often brings new insights, social connection, love, meaning, and personal growth unattained through any other experience.

Caring for someone during end of life is physically, mentally, emotionally, and spiritually demanding. Life's responsibilities (career, household duties, education, care of other family members, and your own personal health and well-being) aren't placed on hold during this time, which means the family of the dying loved one may feel overwhelmed. These feelings can be compounded when involved family members are reluctant to ask for and accept help. It is paramount that family members understand that they must care for their own well-beings to continue to give compassionate support to their loved one nearing end of life. A willing support group is a blessing that we should all seek during this difficult time.

The untiring care provided by hospice professionals must be gratefully acknowledged. These compassionate and skilled professionals play a complex and multifaceted role during very difficult experiences. They too experience a flood of emotions as they struggle to balance meeting the needs of a dying person as human beings and as medical professionals. Their emotional pressures and perpetual brushes with death make it particularly important for them to engage in appropriate self-care and openly acknowledge the complexity of emotions they experience. Medical professionals can also benefit from many of the tips shared throughout this resource.

Each person's dying experience is unique. However, there are shared physical, emotional, mental, and spiritual challenges, many of which essential oils excel at alleviating. The ability of essential oils to affect all aspects of wellness (emotional, mental, physical, and spiritual), their multiple properties (anti-inflammatory, analgesic, antidepressant, anxiolytic, etc.), and the multiple pathways and mechanisms they work therapeutically by are unmatched. Their noninvasive nature, clinically proven efficacy, and wide safety profile makes them ideal solutions during end-of-life care. Their direct connection to areas of the brain that influence mood, emotions, pain, and other psychophysiological functions make them a great solution not only for the person nearing end of life but also for family members and caregivers.

This short reference book is intended to provide concise, brief, and informative information for caregivers, medical professionals, and people nearing death to use essential oils during palliative care—specialized care that improves quality of life and relieves suffering of individuals facing a life-threatening condition, which may also include continuation of curative treatment—and hospice care—a type of palliative care given to people in the final phase of a terminal illness when curative treatment is ceased and the individual has less than six months to live. It is written with the intent and hope that you and those you serve during the end of their lives will be comforted, strengthened, and surrounded by love.

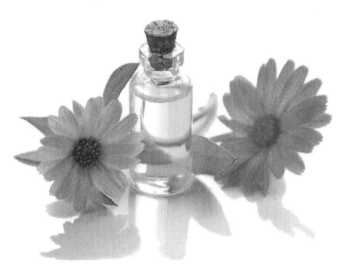

ESSENTIAL OIL QUALITY

First, we need to ensure that the essential oils you use are pure, unadulterated, and high quality. For positive results, you must use a pure and genuine essential oil. Unfortunately, today essential oils are treated much like a commodity. You can purchase essential oils in big-box stores, health food stores, online, and even in airports. However, the quality of one essential oil to another can vary dramatically.

The best essential oils are manufactured using precise standards, which leads to consistent quality, purity, and a preferred chemical profile. The scope of this book isn't to address the topic of essential oil quality comprehensively. You are invited to further explore this subject in one of my many other essential oil books. Instead, I will provide three general guidelines for sourcing a pure essential oil:

1. Be suspicious of essential oils that are offered at significantly lower price than the market. For example, if most lavender essential oils are selling at US$18 to US$28 per 15mL bottle, be cautious of lavender oil selling for less than US$10 for 15mL.

2. Whenever possible, buy your essential oils from a company that provides access to its quality testing for each batch. Gas chromatography mass spectrometry (GC-MS), heavy metals testing, and optical rotation are a few tests that reputable essential oil companies will perform on each batch. Companies willing to provide this data to the end user generally provide higher quality essential oils.

3. Only buy essential oils that list both the common name (peppermint) and the

botanical species (*Mentha piperita*). This will avoid the mistake of purchasing lavandin (*Lavandula × intermedia*) instead of true lavender (*Lavandula angustifolia*).

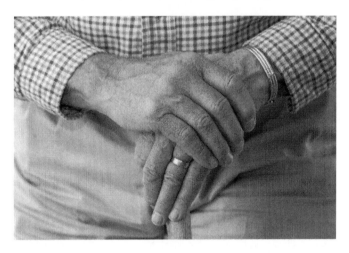

PHYSICAL CHALLENGES

The goal of holistic care for those nearing the end of their lives is to achieve the best quality of life possible for the dying person and his or her loved ones. Passing on to the next life can be quite challenging physically. Research suggests that those nearing the end of their lives experience common physical symptoms that can include physical pain, labored breathing (dyspnea), loss of appetite and weight loss, oral complications, terminal secretions, fatigue, nausea or vomiting, constipation and abdominal pain, insomnia, lymphedema or edema, dehydration, fever, or malnutrition or some combination of these.

Pain

The alleviation of pain and suffering is an essential goal for end-of-life care. Pain is more than a physical experience and is influenced by emotions (anxiety, depression, anger), interpersonal problems (loneliness, family tensions, financial worry), and level of death acceptance (beliefs in the afterlife and hopelessness versus acceptance). There are three main types of physical pain experienced during the final stages of life:

- *Somatic pain*. Pain localized to the skin, soft tissue, muscles, and bones.
- *Visceral pain*. General discomfort or throbbing in the abdomen and internal organs.
- *Neuropathic pain*. A tingling, burning, painful sensation in the extremities.

It is important to recognize the nonverbal signs of pain when caring for a loved one who may be unable to express his or her pain in words. Nonverbal pain cues include

- facial expressions (grimacing, frowning, eyes closed tightly, wrinkled forehead, and distorted expressions);

- body movements (rigid, clenched fists or clenching objects, tense body posture, rocking, restricted movement, and the fetal position);
- vocalizations (moaning, grunting, noisy breathing, sighing);
- changes in mental status or behavior (irritability, aggression, combative, distress, crying, increased confusion, verbally abusive, limited social interaction, and resisting care); and
- changes in routines (appetite change, sudden cessation of common routines, increased sleeping or rest periods).

Two additional characteristics of pain that must be addressed include location and intensity. Intensity is often categorized as a level of 1–10, or the person may be asked to point to a face that identifies the level of pain currently being experienced. Identifying the location and intensity of pain can help the care team manage the pain more effectively.

One of the reasons that essential oils are ideal for pain and discomfort is their dual roles on the physical and mental/emotional aspects of pain. Pain involves the actual raw physical experience (sensory pain) and our perception and emotional reaction (affective pain) to it. These two aspects are closely interrelated. Indeed, people who experience chronic pain are at a greater risk of anxiety and depression disorders.[1] Likewise, hardwired brain defense circuits can be dysregulated when thoughts of pain overwhelm the mind and trigger secondary emotional responses that increase pain and suffering.[2] In other words, individuals may lose the ability to control pain through disruption of key brain circuits until the pain becomes chronic and uninhibited.[3] In addition to modulating key pain and inflammation pathways in the body, essential oils strongly influence the emotions and brain, leading to more complete pain resolution.

Loving touch is one of the most important ways to demonstrate your love and care for your loved one facing end of life. If possible, the essential oil should be applied directly to the area(s) most affected by pain (avoiding sensitive areas near the groin and eyes). If this is not possible because the individual hurts all over and he or she finds touch uncomfortable, a gentle hand or foot massage may be employed. Loving touch can be restorative to key body systems and promote much needed relaxation. The added bonus is that the person giving the massage also receives benefits from the essential oils he or she inhales and absorbs in his or her hands.

Gentle Hand Massage Technique
1. In a 4-ounce (120mL) glass bottle, mix together 15–20 drops of peppermint essential

oil, 10–15 drops of copaiba essential oil, 10–15 drops of bergamot, 8–12 drops of lavender essential oil, and 5–8 drops of ginger essential oil; fill the rest of the bottle with fractionated coconut oil. Shake the bottle well for 30 to 60 seconds to blend.

2. Ensure that the hand of the recipient is free of open wounds and trauma. Do not perform massage if open wounds or trauma is present.

3. Find a position for both you and the recipient to be comfortable during the process.

4. Beginning with the recipient's palm facing down, add some of the essential oil blend to your palm and gently rub it into the back of the recipient's hand all the way up the forearm to the elbow. Continue until the blend is evenly dispersed.

5. Starting at the wrist area, use your thumbs to glide from the center of the back of the hand out over the edge of the hand three times (dividing the area from the wrist to the knuckles in thirds or fourths) until you reach the fingers. Repeat this step three times down the hand.

6. Then, starting at the wrist, gently glide down over each finger individually until you move off the fingertips.

7. Turn the recipient's hand over so the palm faces up and add some of the essential oil

blend to your palm. Gently rub the essential oil into the recipient's palm and forearm.

8. With your thumbs near the wrist, perform circular movements downward from the wrist to each finger, finishing by stroking down each finger and off the fingertip. Repeat this step three times.

9. Finish by performing a thumb walk down the midline of the palm. Repeat three times.

10. Repeat the procedure on the recipient's other hand.

Watch a video demonstration of the Gentle Hand Massage at: https://youtu.be/ShT8xjXqcTA.

Gentle Foot Massage Technique

1. In a 4-ounce (120mL) glass bottle, mix together 15–20 drops of peppermint essential oil, 10–15 drops of copaiba essential oil, 10–15 drops of bergamot, 8–12 drops of lavender essential oil, and 5–8 drops of ginger essential oil; fill the rest of the bottle with fractionated coconut oil. Shake the bottle well for 30 to 60 seconds to blend.

2. Ensure that the foot of the recipient is free of open wounds and trauma. Do not perform massage if open wounds or trauma is present.

3. Find a position for both you and the recipient to be comfortable during the process.

4. Add some of the essential oil blend to the palm of your hand and gently rub it into the bottom of the recipient's foot up the calf and to the knee (if possible; if not continue up the calve as far as possible). Continue until the blend is evenly dispersed.
5. Begin with a thumb walk on the midline of the foot from the heel to the ball ensuring your thumb walk continues horizontally under each toe. Repeat this action three times.
6. Starting with your thumbs at the center of the heel, glide from the midline of the foot to the edges with your thumbs until you reach the ball of the foot. Repeat this action three times.
7. Finish by rubbing the entire foot with your palm and gently pulling on each toe.
8. Repeat the procedure on the recipient's other foot.

Watch a video demonstration of the Gentle Foot Massage at: https://youtu.be/80exIGtZcTI.

Loss of Appetite, Weight Loss, and Malnutrition
Chronic and systemic illness—such as cancer, AIDS, heart failure—may cause wasting syndromes such as anorexia (loss of appetite) and cachexia (body mass loss or weight loss). Fatigue and the appearance of malnutrition are often the result. However, the significant weight loss suffered by people nearing the end of life is not entirely attributed to decreased

caloric intake. Cachexia should be viewed as a larger set of gastrointestinal and constitutional disorders associated with the disease (condition) process and not always as reversible by increased calorie consumption. While distressing symptoms, gentle encouragement, patience, and understanding should prevail among caregivers.

Loss of appetite is one of the most commonly reported concerns of those caring for a loved one who is dying. Providing food to loved ones is a symbolic gesture of nurturing and love. Caregivers may feel as if they have failed their loved one when he or she refuses to eat. This destructive notion couldn't be further from the truth.

People nearing the end of life commonly have decreased appetite and shouldn't be forced to eat. Loss of appetite is a normal and natural part of the dying process. As death nears, the body's metabolism slows down and less nutrition is required. Medications may also change eating habits and preferences. In addition, increased weakness and drowsiness makes swallowing and digesting food more difficult. In fact, eating may divert energy to the digestive process and place more strain on the rest of the body. This doesn't mean your loved one should be deprived of food, but he or she should be permitted to eat when he or she feels up to it and when physically possible with aspiration risk.

Some cases of anorexia and cachexia may be reversible, including those caused by chronic pain, oral health (dryness, mucositis—painful inflammation and sores of the mucous membranes caused by chemo or radiotherapy), constipation, and gastroesophageal reflux.

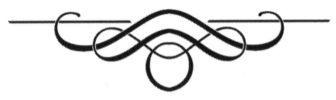

Nutritional support can be beneficial—reduce deterioration, improve quality of life, and evasion of the emotional experience of "starving the loved one to death"—if a little can be eaten. Ultimately, your loved one's desire for food and water—and his or her level of awareness and ability to eat or drink—should be the chief guide in determining nutrition and hydration requirements.

Despite the appearance of malnutrition, these wasting syndromes are most often caused by the disease causing the death of your loved one and not generally reversible with improved nutrition.

Research suggests that aggressive attempts to nourish terminally ill individuals is of little benefit and may actually cause more harm or discomfort (increased body fat, nausea, vomiting, edema, bowel and bladder incontinence, and bleeding).[4,5,6,7,8,9,10] Cachexia should therefore be expected as a consequence of the disease and dying process and not considered inadequate care and nutrition.

A better approach to these wasting syndromes is to focus on strategies that alleviate symptoms and increase comfort. The following are tips to help do so:

- Moisten your loved one's lips and mouth with a clean oral-care sponge frequently if dryness is a symptom. Any liquid on the sponge will do. The lips can be moistened with a natural lip balm as well. Indeed, some evidence suggests that meticulous mouth care may be more important than hydration.[11,12]
- Provide "comfort" or favorite foods that will likely give your loved one enjoyment when requested.
- Offer small frequent meals when your loved one has the most energy and the least pain.
- Don't pressure your loved one to eat. Instead, maintain a relaxed tone around eating, with an emphasis on enjoyment.

- Serve beverages (water, warm herbal teas, coconut water) between meals to encourage feelings of fullness and reduce hunger.
- Consider combining meals with pleasurable activities like company of friends and family, favorite music, or favorite movies.
- Consider providing *Moringa oleifera* leaf in beverage form. The edible parts of this tree (leaves, fruit, and seed) contain a wide variety (over ninety nutrients total) of vitamins, minerals, amino acids, and phytocompounds. This infusion of nutrients can strengthen the cells and help your loved one endure the challenges of dying.
- Use bendable or shorter straws if drawing liquids is difficult.
- Use easy-to-handle dishware, flatware, and glasses.

In addition to the above tips, essential oils may be used to improve appetite if appropriate. Odors have been used for centuries to affect eating behaviors in humans and to influence desire for food. Commonly used essential oils include bergamot, lemon, lime, orange, fennel, lavender, caraway, cardamom, coriander, tarragon, peppermint, clove, and cumin. Although human clinical research regarding the appetite-enhancing effects of essential oils is lacking, some preclinical research suggests they do increase appetite. Inhalation of lavender essential oil has proven to enhance appetite in a preclinical model.[13] Scientists have also observed essential oils that contain phenylpropanoids (i.e., trans-cinnamaldehyde, eugenol, trans-anethole) increase appetite. Clove, cinnamon, anise, and fennel are four essential oils often rich in phenylpropanoids. Components of curry oil (trans-cinnamaldehyde, trans-anethole, and eugenol) showed appetite-enhancing effects in mice.[14,15] Emerging preclinical research suggests that odors can influence pathways involved in appetite regulation and are therefore promising solutions for appetite dysregulation.

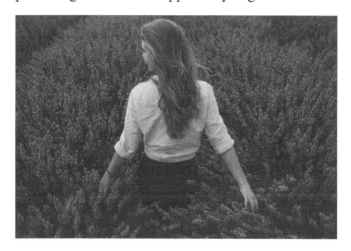

Based on this research and traditional usage, it may be beneficial to inhale essential oils like cinnamon, clove, lavender, anise, and fennel to improve the desire for food. Your loved one should be given a few essential oils to choose from to determine a pleasing aroma because the like or dislike of aromas is subjective. Once a desirable essential oil—or combination of essential oils—is selected, diffuse the oil approximately thirty minutes before meal or snack time. Alternately, place a few drops on a cotton ball and place it near your loved one about thirty minutes before offering food. At the very least, the inhalation of essential oils can be a pleasing sensation and could perhaps provide supplementary benefits such as mood improvement.

Oral Complications
Dry mouth (xerostomia), candida, difficulty swallowing (dysphagia), stomatitis (painful swelling and sores inside the mouth), and mucositis are common in individuals nearing the end of their lives. The mouth is frequently the first site that manifests the side effects of treatment, or it may be compromised directly by advanced disease. Oral complications that arise during the end of life can impact quality of life because oral health is vital to communication, eating, and swallowing. Oral health must therefore not be overlooked by caregivers of individuals approaching death.

Dry mouth can be managed through recurrent moistening of the oral cavity with a clean and wet oral-care sponge. Frequent sips of water and the use of a humidifier are also valuable. Bitter and sour flavors may increase salivation, but don't overdo it. Xylitol-based gums, candies, and mints can stimulate natural saliva production and promote oral health. Lozenges naturally sweetened with honey and essential oils can also provide relief from dry mouth. Even sucking on a lemon slice may be helpful. Candies, gum, mints, and lozenges should be used only when appropriate based on the person's current state of health and ability to use these products without choking. These simple solutions can go a long way to improve oral health and your loved one's quality of life.

Stomatitis is inflammation of the mucous membranes (thin skin coverings on the inside of the surface of the mouth) in the oral cavity, with or without ulcers. The membranes produce the protective mucus and lining of the digestive system from the mouth to the anus. Stomatitis is typically a result of poor oral hygiene or damage to the mucous membranes. It can also be caused by chemotherapy, radiotherapy, breathing through the mouth, or clogged nasal passages. Timely management of stomatitis can improve quality of life.

If you notice bad breath or your loved one complains of an unpleasant taste, it may be a sign that the oral cavity contains candida. Candida is a genus of yeasts (*Candida albicans* being the most common species) that normally exists in the gut, mucous membranes, on the skin, and in the vagina. It isn't a problem under normal circumstances where it coexists with bacteria in the body. But it can wreak havoc throughout the body when it grows and overpopulates the digestive tract or vagina.

Oropharyngeal candidiasis (oral thrush) is a condition characterized by white patches in the mouth, inner cheeks, throat, tongue, and palate. It may also cause mouth pain. Be aware that some medications can cause thrush (corticosteroids, antibiotics, and chemotherapy) and people with HIV, cancer, uncontrolled diabetes, and smokers have an increased risk of thrush. Antifungal mouthwashes are most commonly used to treat oral thrush, but natural solutions are also helpful.

Brushing at least twice daily is important but may be too painful with a mouth full of sores. If brushing isn't an option, swab the mouth with toothette swabs (perhaps with a small amount of alcohol-free mouthwash and a drop of tea tree essential oil) at least twice daily. Alcohol-free (alcohol dries the mouth) and natural mouthwashes can also be helpful, particularly if you add a drop of tea tree essential oil to each use of the mouthwash.[16] Other essential oils that may be useful for oral care include geranium, lavender, and peppermint, possibly in a blend with tea tree.[17] Regular oral care will improve oral cleanliness and quality of life.

To address oral pain or discomfort, consider using clove and copaiba essential oils. Clove, or its primary constituent eugenol, has a long history of use in oral care. It acts as a topical analgesic (pain reliever). Copaiba has been used for pain and inflammation among Amazonian tribes for decades. Combining the two makes an effective oral pain solution. In a 5mL bottle, combine 5 drops each of clove and copaiba essential oil. Fill the rest of the bottle with fractionated coconut oil. Apply a drop or two of this mixture to affected areas as needed.

Difficulty swallowing is also common among individuals nearing end of life. It can be both frustrating and frightening for the caregiver. Signs to watch for include "cheeking" foods instead of swallowing, prolonged time to eat, food or beverages leaking out of the mouth, and aspiration (inhaling small food particles into the lungs). Feeding tubes may be presented as an option if dysphagia is a problem, but these are invasive and have limited success. With some patience and the right strategies, you may be able to improve swallowing naturally.

Interestingly, clinical research suggests that inhalation of black pepper essential oil may relieve dysphagia. Japanese scientists evaluated olfactory stimulation using black pepper in elderly individuals who experienced difficulty swallowing after a stroke. Participants inhaled 100 mcL (about 2 to 3 drops depending on the orifice reducer) of black pepper essential oil from a paper stick for one minute prior to each meal. What the researchers found was that the black pepper oil improved swallowing reflexes by activating the insular and orbitofrontal areas of the brain.[18] Given the noninvasive nature of inhaling black pepper essential oil, it makes sense to add 2 to 3 drops to a cotton ball and have your loved one inhale it for a minute prior to each meal to improve dysphagia.

In addition to black pepper essential oil inhalation, you can consider the following strategies:

- Chop or blend the food into a puree or smoothie.
- Provide smaller meals.
- Avoid dry, crumbly foods (like crackers).
- Avoid sticky foods (like peanut butter).

Terminal Secretions

Terminal secretions originating from the respiratory system are also a frequent occurrence among the imminently dying person.[19] The majority of dying individuals pass to the next life within forty-eight hours after the occurrence of respiratory secretions and the "death rattle"—a gurgling noise heard in a dying person's throat.[20] Terminal secretions are thought to be caused by pooled respiratory secretions that occur as the person becomes weaker and loses the ability to cough or swallow normally. It is a distressing noise and symptom that family members frequently express concern over.

Unfortunately, antisecretory medications—atropine, glycopyrrolate, Hyoscine, Buscopan—are not always effective (especially if not administered very soon after the symptoms begin), and frequent suctioning can be uncomfortable to the dying individual. In addition, secretions are frequently below the larynx and inaccessible to suction. Frequent suctioning should be discouraged unless copious frothing or thick mucus, blood, or other fluid is present in the mouth. It should be emphasized to loved ones distressed over the noise and secretions that this is a normal part of the dying process. Aspiration of secretions should be prevented by repositioning your loved one on his or her back or side with the head slightly raised to encourage drainage and decrease pooling of secretions. Good mouth care should be continued and overhydration avoided.

The drugs used to reduce terminal secretions are anticholinergics (agents that block the action of acetylcholine, which is a neurotransmitter and chemical messenger involved in parasympathetic nerve impulses). Some essential oils (oregano, thyme, bergamot, clove, lemon, lime, marjoram, etc.) also act as anticholinergics but are not likely to work topically or aromatically.[21] Instead, these essential oils may need to be given sublingually or on the tongue to attempt to limit terminal secretions. Many of these essential oils would be quite "warm" if applied directly in the oil, which limits the options to the citrus essential oils. If the secretions are problematic or overly troubling, it may be worth adding one drop of bergamot, lemon, or lime essential oil onto or under the tongue every thirty minutes for up to four doses, then every two to four hours thereafter.

Fatigue

Fatigue (a persistent state of tiredness that is not relieved by rest or sleep) is among the most commonly reported symptoms experienced by individuals nearing the end of life. Over time, your loved one will become increasingly tired and weak. This fatigue gradually increases until it becomes unconsciousness in many terminally ill individuals. Fatigue is multidimensional and causes physical, emotional, and cognitive difficulties.

Because fatigue is determined by both physical and psychological factors, essential oils are again an ideal solution. Japanese scientists investigated the benefits of essential oils combined with the principles of reflexology in people with advanced cancer (a group that commonly experiences fatigue). The fatigued individuals included in the study received a foot soak with lavender for three minutes, followed by reflexology with lavender diluted in jojoba oil. Lavender's relaxing properties are well-known, but interestingly in this case, the lavender foot soak and reflexology effectively relieved fatigue.[22] The results underscore the adaptability of essential oils to the individual's needs.

To simulate the study design, fill a pan with comfortably warm water. Add two to three drops of lavender essential oil to one-half cup of Epsom salts and mix in the warm water. Allow your loved one to soak his or her feet in the foot soak for up to twenty minutes—adding warm water as necessary to maintain a comfortable temperature. After twenty minutes, dry his or her feet and follow the directions for the gentle foot massage technique, using one drop of lavender in 1–2mL of fractionated coconut oil for each foot. Add orange or tangerine essential oils for improved aroma if desired.

It may also be helpful to diffuse a mixture of peppermint, basil, and helichrysum. These essential oils have proven effective in reducing mental exhaustion in clinical research.[23] Alternately, place one to two drops of peppermint on a cotton ball and allow your loved one to inhale the peppermint as needed.

Nausea and Vomiting
Feeling nauseous is uncomfortable and significantly disrupts normal daily activities. Effective

management of nausea and vomiting can significantly improve quality of life in those nearing end of life. Although distressing, nausea and vomiting appears to occur less frequently than originally believed (43 percent in late-stage AIDS, 30 percent in end-stage kidney disease, 17 percent during heart failure, and only 6 percent of people suffering from terminal cancer).[24] Other reports suggest it is far more prevalent—62 percent in cancer patients and 40 percent among those in their last six weeks of life.[25] Those still undergoing treatment, such as chemotherapy, are more likely to experience nausea and vomiting than those whose treatment has ended. Even if it is less common, it can be debilitating, and so you and your loved one should be prepared to handle it if it occurs.

Nausea and vomiting is a complex process that involves several pathways and receptors:

1) **The vomiting center**. Located in the brainstem and involves histamine (H1), acetylcholine (ACh), and 5-hydroxytryptamine 2 (5-HT2) receptors.

2) **The chemoreceptor trigger zone**. Not protected by a blood-brain barrier, this area of the brain enables various drugs, toxins, and metabolites to access its dopamine (D2) and 5-HT3 receptors.

3) **The cerebral cortex**. This is the outer layer of the cerebral hemispheres. It contains about twenty billion neurons, which carry out the highest levels of cognitive functioning. The cerebral cortex contains multiple receptors, including receptors in the meninges that are sensitive to changes in intracranial pressure.
4) **The vestibular system**. This system monitors information about motion, spatial orientation, and equilibrium. Changes in movement or conditions involving the inner ear may stimulate ACh and H1 receptors and cause nausea and vomiting.
5) **Gut**. 5-HT3 receptors in the gut may be triggered by bacteria, toxins, drugs, and radiotherapy. The linings of visceral organs also contain H1 and ACh receptors that can cause nausea/vomiting when stimulated.

Blocking these receptor sites is the primary target of drug therapies to reduce nausea and vomiting.

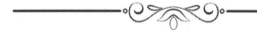

Assessing possible causes of nausea and vomiting is key to its management. If it occurs after meals, disordered or delayed gastric emptying (gastric stasis) may be the cause. Movement that triggers symptoms suggests vestibular disorder. If symptoms are aggravated by lying flat, meningeal irritation or increased intracranial pressure may be the source.

The timing of symptoms in relation to drug administration should also be considered.

Possible Cause	Signs and Symptoms
Meningeal irritation	• Headache and nausea when lying flat • Focal neurological deficits: impairments of central nervous system function that affects a specific region of the body (i.e., weakness of one limb) • Papilledema (optic disk swelling due to increased intracranial pressure) • CT- and MRI-scan confirmation (may be performed during palliative care, not normally performed for those under hospice care)
Bowel obstruction	• Abdominal pain • Gradual onset • Profuse vomiting if the obstruction is high
Gastric stasis	• Feeling of fullness or early satiety

	• Upper central region abdominal pain • Hiccups • Acid reflux • Little nausea • Symptoms are relieved after vomiting
Chemically caused	• Symptoms coincide with starting medication • Confusion • Drowsiness
Anxiety related	• Symptoms occur with other signs of stress • After ruling out other causes
Movement related	• Vestibular disorder • Opioids recently introduced or dosage increased

Essential oils can be effective in relieving nausea and vomiting simply through inhalation. The most commonly used essential oils for nausea and vomiting include peppermint, spearmint, ginger, and lemon. To create a blend for nausea and vomiting, combine 50 drops each of peppermint and spearmint, 35 drops of lemon, and 15 drops of ginger in a 5mL bottle. Shake well. Inhale directly from the bottle, or add a few drops to a cotton ball, and inhale as needed.

Constipation

End-of-life constipation is common and can be caused by multiple factors (long-term use of opioids, reduced mobility, reduced fluid intake, tumors that obstruct or compress the bowel, and neurological disease). The symptoms include abdominal discomfort or distention, bloating, gas, hard stools, straining during a bowel movement, and a feeling of incomplete bowel emptying after a bowel movement. As constipation can affect your loved one's quality of life, steps should be taken to promote regular bowel movements when safe, practical, and reasonable.

It should be noted that constipation is less of a concern as your loved one approaches his or her final days. It is not uncommon for individuals very close to death to go several days without a bowel movement; however, hospice professionals may be instructed to administer a suppository if more than three days have passed since a bowel movement. Your loved one's comfort should be the primary guiding factor as to whether intervention is necessary.

One of the most effective remedies for constipation is senna leaf tea. This is an option as long as your loved one is not experiencing bowel obstruction, acute intestinal inflammation (Crohn's disease or ulcerative colitis), stomach inflammation, or hemorrhoids. Depending on the strength of the tea and how much senna it contains, it could cause diarrhea, so caution is advised if your loved one has never used senna tea before.

Abdominal massage has been used to relieve constipation since the nineteenth century. It effectively relieves constipation by stimulating peristalsis (the rhythmic muscular contraction of the bowels), increasing the speed at which food travels through the digestive tract, and by increasing bowel-movement frequency. Abdominal massage is pleasant, relaxing, and enhances both communication and social interaction of the two parties involved.[26] In addition, abdominal massage alleviates pain and discomfort associated with constipation. With virtually no adverse effects, abdominal massage is a leading option to relieve constipation.

While abdominal massage alone is effective, incorporating specific essential oils into the massage may be even more effective. Sluggish bowels are frequently reported among the elderly, and so Korean researchers set out to investigate the effects of an abdominal massage with essential oil for constipation in elderly individuals. What they found was that abdominal massage with rosemary, lemon, and peppermint essential oils relieved constipation.[27]

Remarkably, the bowel benefits of the essential oil massage lasted for two weeks.

The researchers created a massage blend of three parts rosemary, four parts lemon, and two parts peppermint essential oil in a mixture of three parts sweet almond oil and one part jojoba oil. The final mixture was 3 percent (about three drops of the blend of essential oils per 5mL of the blended carrier oil). The abdominal massage consisted of circular, clockwise movements along the line of the colon with the hands for five to ten minutes. This action glides over the ascending, transverse, descending, and sigmoid colon. The massage as performed for a period of 5–10 minutes, preferably 30 minutes.

Abdominal Massage Technique

1. Do not perform abdominal massage if intestinal obstruction, abdominal mass, intestinal bleeding, or hernia exists.
2. In a 15mL bottle, add four drops of lemon essential oil, three drops of rosemary essential oil, and two drops of peppermint essential oil. For ease, use only fractionated coconut oil to fill the rest of the bottle. Shake well to blend.
3. Massage should ideally be performed after a meal. It should be of gentle to moderate pressure and performed daily until bowel movement occurs.

4. Place approximately 5mL of the mixture in your palm and spread over the recipient's lower abdominal region around the belly button.

5. Beginning in the lower right area of the recipient's abdomen, massage up the right side, across the top, and down the left side of the abdomen (around the belly button) in a circular motion. Repeat this motion for at least five to ten minutes and up to thirty minutes.

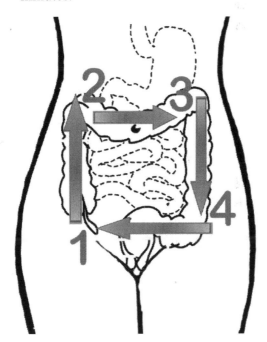

Insomnia

Sleep patterns change during the aging process. Older adults often have difficulty falling asleep and staying asleep. In addition, they tend to get insufficient time in the deep sleep stage of the sleep cycle, leaving them tired and groggy despite a full night's sleep. Those nearing the end of their lives similarly experience problems initiating or maintaining sleep.

Disturbed or impaired sleep can leave your loved one feeling nonrestored and unrefreshed. And since over sixty percent of people in palliative care (and it can be expected that hospice care shares this statistic) experience insomnia, it can dramatically affect quality of life.[28,29] Poor sleep can lead to a vicious cycle that coexists with and often exacerbates other symptoms such as pain and mood disturbances.

Some causes of insomnia that should be addressed include pain that interferes with restful sleep, difficulty breathing (which may be worse when lying down), and digestive problems (i.e., acid reflux).

Inhalation of aromatic scents was believed to be practiced anciently to promote relaxation and improve sleep. Three leading essential oils to consider to improve sleep quality include lavender, vetiver, and Roman chamomile.

Lavender has been investigated in multiple clinical studies evaluating sleep quality. Inhalation of lavender oil directly from a glass bottle between the hours of 10:00 p.m. and 6:00 a.m. improved the sleep quality of individuals in a hospital intermediate care unit.[30] Dementia and Alzheimer's disease impacts the brain in a way that causes sleep disturbances. Diffusion of lavender oil during sleeping hours reduced insomnia and anxiety among people with dementia living in nursing homes.[31] Healthy individuals experienced increased deep sleep when lavender was inhaled intermittently while sleeping (such as a diffuser set to mist for short periods followed by periods of rest).[32] Another small study found that lavender oil inhalation reduced mild insomnia.[33] Lavender has proven itself time and time again as an effective solution for sleep disturbances.

Lavender pairs well with other essential oils to enhance the benefits of aromatherapy. One study tested the benefits of a hand massage with lavender and bergamot essential oil (10 drops of each in 100 mL of jojoba carrier oil) on fatigue and sleeping among hospice patients. The hand massage was performed for ten minutes prior to sleeping time, once daily for five days. The aromatherapy massage slightly improved their quality of sleep and reduced fatigue when compared to those who received a hand massage with jojoba oil alone.[34] The results may have improved if the researchers had used a higher concentration of essential oil (perhaps 3 percent).

GABA (gamma-aminobutyric acid) is a calming neurotransmitter that dampens nerve activity. People with insomnia frequently have reduced levels of GABA, which is why some sleeping pills act by improving the ability of GABA to bind to brain receptors. Vetiver can increase GABA levels and the activity of GABA in the brain to promote restful sleep.[35,36,37,38] The aromatic influence of vetiver on the brain means your loved one can relax and sleep without grogginess in the morning.

As previously mentioned, difficulty breathing may cause insomnia. Interestingly, clinical research suggests that both lavender and vetiver essential oils improve breathing patterns during sleep.[39] Since they also aid sleep quality, they are ideal essential oils for those nearing the end of their lives who have trouble sleeping.

If your loved one is having trouble sleeping during or after cancer treatment, he or she is not alone. Some experts estimate that nearly half of all cancer patients don't sleep well. Emotional distress is the primary reason those with cancer have sleep difficulties. One study reported that inhalation of blends of either bergamot and sandalwood or another blend with frankincense, tangerine, and lavender essential oils improved sleep quality among people with cancer.[40]

This effect may be due to the relaxing and emotionally balancing effects of the essential oils used, therefore, reducing the primary cause of insomnia among cancer patients—emotional distress.

Select one or more of the above essential oils that your loved one finds pleasing. Once selected, you can diffuse several drops (five to ten) in a diffuser on intermittent, add up to 3 drops to a cotton ball and place near your loved one, or place a few drops in a glass near him or her. In addition, you could mix two or three drops of your loved one's chosen oils into some carrier oil and use the gentle hand or foot massage technique approximately 15 minutes before bedtime. Essential oils may be the key to a good night's sleep and much needed recuperation.

Labored Breathing or Shortness of Breath (Dyspnea)

Labored or noisy breathing and coughing are commonly reported in people nearing the end of life due to the accumulation of fluids in the throat (see the Terminal Secretions section in this book for more information). Evidence suggests that 70 percent of people in their last six weeks of life experience dyspnea.[41] This can produce anxiety in both the dying individual and the caregiver.

Your loved one may describe this as shortness of breath, tightness in the chest, or the feeling of not getting enough air. Dyspnea may occur as a consequence of the disease, infection (pneumonia), chemotherapy drug side effect, and even anxiety.

Some practical measures to take for your loved one include the following:

- Keep the room cool.
- Provide good air movement near him or her.
- Minimize his or her exertion or anxiety.
- Administration of oxygen.
- Position your loved one sitting with his or her body leaning forward and arms resting on a table.

Some of the most prized essential oils for the respiratory system include eucalyptus (*Eucalyptus globulus, Eucalyptus radiata*), peppermint, and myrtle. Frankincense is balancing to the respiratory system and often used to regulate irregular breathing. Other beneficial respiratory oils include spruce, balsam fir, pine, sandalwood, ravintsara (1,8-cineole type), cajeput, and oregano. In addition, calming oils like lavender, Roman chamomile, citrus oils, and frankincense may reduce anxiety-related dyspnea.

Diffusion with a nebulizing (atomizing) essential oil diffuser is the most direct way to inhale essential oils. This technology disperses millions of undiluted essential oil microparticles into the air, which are taken into the lungs. If a nebulizing diffuser is not available, use an ultrasonic diffuser or simply add a few drops to some hot water in a bowl and place near your loved one. Combinations of the above mentioned essential oils are likely to be more effective than single oils alone.

Fever

Your loved one may or may not experience a fever, but it is common nearer to death. Indeed, a low-grade fever is considered by many hospice professionals as part of the dying process. A clinically significant fever is considered a body temperature over 100.4˚F (38˚C). An elevated temperature can be due to an infection, but is more likely the result of changes in metabolism.

Mild fevers that don't seem to bother your loved one can be managed with tepid sponge baths and essential oils. A clean sponge or washcloth dipped in tepid water can be applied across the trunk, arms, and legs for several minutes. A drop or two of peppermint essential oil may be added to the tepid water, but do not apply the sponge near the eyes if you do so. Another option is to mix two to three drops of peppermint essential oil in 5 mL of carrier oil, then apply a small amount of this mixture to the feet or spine. These strategies can promote cooling if your loved one is bothered by an elevated temperature.

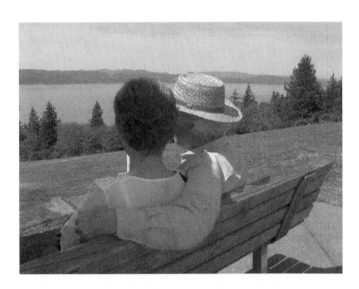

EMOTIONAL CHALLENGES

Anxiety, Grief, and Depression

It is normal to feel some amount of anxiety, grief, or depression when nearing the end of life. These feelings are shared by friends and loved ones of the person dying. Caregivers and palliative care/hospice professionals are strongly encouraged to incorporate appropriate recommendations in this section to care for their emotional and mental well-being.

The loss of functionality (strength to get around, eating, or other enjoyable activities) by your loved one may contribute to negative emotions. Another reason negative emotions may be present include family and loved ones who seem distant as they struggle to come to terms with the impending death. The dying individual may also be concerned about being a burden to others, adding to his or her emotional grief. Since grief is an almost universal feeling for the individual dying and his or her loved ones, it is something you can work together to overcome.

It is noteworthy that a significant number of family members caring for terminally ill loved ones experience anxiety or depression. Research suggests that nearly one-quarter of those caring for the terminally ill experience moderate to severe depression and a greater number (nearly one-third) report moderate to severe anxiety symptoms.[42] This highlights the need to provide emotional care for the whole family, caregivers, and hospice professionals, not just the one nearing end of life.

Talking to someone you trust—loved one, dear friend, or ecclesiastical leader—can help you process these feelings. It certainly isn't healthy to bottle up the emotions and attempt to handle them alone. Although one of the most painful parts of dying, overcoming grief is tremendously healing. Once you do this, you may feel a burden has been lifted, which allows you to focus on other physical and emotional tasks that are part of the end of life.

A long history of use and mounting scientific evidence suggests that essential oils excel in relieving mood disturbances. Several clinical studies have investigated the effects of aromatherapy for mood disturbances and anxiety associated with dying.

Understanding that nurses caring for those nearing death use massage and essential oils more frequently, a researcher from the University of Liverpool attempted to assess whether this practice improved patient quality of life. The participants in the study received three full-body massages over the course of three weeks, with or without (control group) Roman chamomile essential oil. Significant improvements in physical and psychological symptoms were realized among people nearing the end of life who received full-body massages with Roman chamomile.[43] The study author concluded that massage with Roman chamomile essential oil is "beneficial in reducing anxiety, tension, pain, and depression."

A few years later the same researcher teamed with other scientists to further investigate massage with Roman chamomile essential oil. Both massage groups (with and without Roman chamomile) experienced decreased anxiety levels. However, only the group that received massage with Roman chamomile achieved significant improvements in psychological state and quality of life, and reductions in severe physical and psychological symptoms.[44] The conclusion drawn was that the combination of essential oil and massage enhances improvements in physical and psychological symptoms, as well as overall quality of life, associated with end of life.

Korean researchers evaluated the benefits of essential oil hand massage with lavender and frankincense essential oil. The two oils were blended in sweet almond carrier oil and diluted to a 3 percent to 5 percent concentration. For those receiving chemotherapy, the concentration was diluted to 1.5 percent. The essential oil hand massage was performed once daily for seven days and for five minutes on each hand. Massage was usually performed between the hours of 2:00 p.m. and 5:00 p.m. What the researchers found was that the essential oil hand massage positively affected depression and pain.[45]

Another study also investigated the benefits of lavender essential oil, only this study used an inhalation method. Three groups were included in the study: 1) no treatment (control); 2) water humidification only; and 3) three percent humidified lavender oil inhalation. Humidified lavender oil was inhaled for sixty minutes [the humidified water (group 2) was inhaled for the same time]. The researchers measured vital signs as well as pain, anxiety, depression, and sense of well-being a day before inhalation, the day of inhalation, and a day after inhalation. Interestingly, both the humidified water and the humidified lavender groups experienced positive, although slight, effects on blood pressure and pulse, pain, anxiety, depression, and sense of well-being.[46] The results suggest that inhalation of humidified water or lavender are equally effective and indicate that massage with essential oil may be more effective than inhalation only.

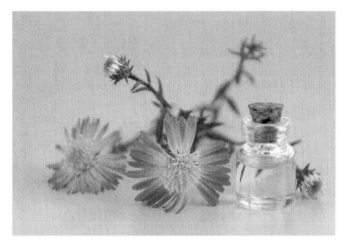

Each of the essential oils used in the studies provides both physical and psychological benefits. They are well-known for their pain-relieving and mood-balancing effects, making them excellent choices for people nearing the end of life. By using Roman chamomile, frankincense, or lavender essential oil, you can provide for your loved one's physical, mental, and emotional care.

Full-body massages are not always practical for individuals nearing the end of life. However, you can perform the gentle hand or foot massage techniques with any of the above mentioned essential oils, or blends that include them. One of my personal favorite blends for grief is one I formulated (known as Embolden) that contains copaiba, Atlas cedarwood, frankincense (*Boswellia carterii*), rosemary, lavender, geranium, and German chamomile.

Fear

People are often afraid to die. Fear may be related to several aspects of dying. They may be concerned about the possibility of a next life. They may fear suffering and pain. Or they may have regrets and consternation that their lives had no meaning or purpose. These are all common reasons that people fear death that can be lessened with appropriate care.

A fear of the next life is often deep-seated in religious and cultural beliefs. Death need not be frightening. Death is a part of life. This text is not the place to discuss religion or the afterlife, nor the varying beliefs in it, but those with the strongest faith are best able to face death without fear. A compassionate ecclesiastical leader may be of benefit for those who fear the next life. In addition, the dying person's loved ones can be a huge factor in providing hope.

One of the most important ways to reassure your loved one who fears the pain and discomfort associated with death is to take measures to minimize these physical symptoms. Comfort your loved one by helping him or her understand that he or she will experience little or no pain unless this is what he or she chooses. At the very least, assure your loved one that the care team will do everything possible to minimize the pain he or she feels and keep him or her comfortable.

In some circumstances, drugs are insufficient to dull pain sufficiently. This is why it is important to not chase pain, meaning don't forgo the necessary use of pain medications or essential oils or both early in the care process. It is difficult to reverse pain once severe pain has set in without powerful narcotics like morphine.

A willingness to experience pain may be spiritually or religiously related. Some individuals believe that enduring pain is ennobling. It may be considered earned punishment for sin or bad behavior. Others consider it a form of spiritual purification, while some individuals request to cross over to the next life with a clear mind unaltered by pain medications. In the end, your loved one's wishes on how pain is managed should be considered paramount.

If the fear is for the loved ones who will be left behind, a detailed plan should be made for their future care. This can help your loved one understand that everything will be okay and that loved ones left behind will be cared for. Give the loved one audible permission to let go and pass, confirming that those left behind will be fine.

Some individuals find the following phrases empowering and healing: "I'm sorry," "Please forgive me," "I love you," and "Thank you." These words embody repentance, forgiveness, gratitude, and love and provide peace and comfort for both the dying individual and his or her caregivers.

Regrets about the past and a lack of meaning or purpose in the life lived is more challenging. Efforts should be made to shift your loved one's focus to the life he or she lived and the positive impact he or she had in other's lives. Sharing of personal stories and situations when your loved one made a positive impact should be communicated whenever possible.

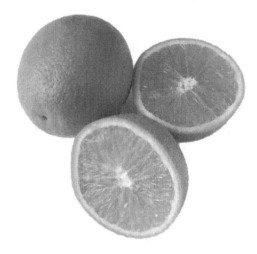

Some essential oils that have been used to reduce fear include black pepper, Roman chamomile, sweet orange, cedarwood (Atlas, Texas, or Virginia), ylang ylang, lavender, lemon, and vetiver. Allow your loved one to choose any of these essential oils or a blend that contains them and inhale as necessary to push away feelings of fear. They can also be incorporated into gentle hand and foot massages.

Social Withdrawal
During your loved one's last days, he or she may desire to decrease social interactions or lose interest in the people around him or her. Understand that withdrawal is not personal; it is a natural part of the dying process. You should strive to continue meaningful communication and provide gentle, affectionate touches to your loved one, especially during required interaction times (medications, mealtimes).

Social withdrawal can be managed much the same as grief, anxiety, and depression. Essential oils are multitarget, multimechanism complex molecules that can affect myriad physical and psychological functions. As such, the powerhouses of lavender, Roman chamomile, and frankincense may also be useful if social withdrawal is not a symptom of the body shutting down. Diffusing essential oils as well as gentle massages may be comforting.

Anger

Many people don't feel ready to die, leading to feelings of anger. This is especially true for those who near death sooner than they expected—feeling cheated of a longer life. An early death is undeserved, and you and your loved one have every right to be mad. Unfortunately, anger is not constructive and only harmful as it is often directed at those we love most.

Like with social withdrawal, diffusing essential oils or soothing massages can be helpful to release anger. German chamomile, Roman chamomile, lavender, helichrysum, melissa, peppermint, pine, vetiver, and mandarin essential oils are all common essential oils utilized to combat anger.

Guilt and Regret

Feeling guilty for being a "burden" to family is a frequent occurrence. Guilt about leaving loved ones behind is also common. Your loved one may also feel regret and wish he or she could have done something differently during his or her lifetime. Sadly, guilt and regret won't ease any burdens and will only make your loved one feel bad.

If possible, your loved one should be encouraged to "let it go" and focus his or her remaining days not feeling guilty about things that are no longer within his or her control. The past can't be changed, but apologies and forgiveness—of self and others—may provide much needed emotional comfort and relief.

Cypress, juniper berry (*Juniperus communis*), sandalwood, thyme, and cardamom essential oils are frequently mentioned to reduce feelings of guilt and regret. Diffuse or massage any of them into the hands following the gentle hand massage instructions.

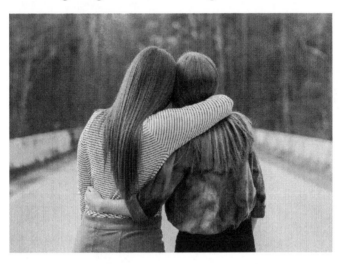

MENTAL CHALLENGES

Delirium

Delirium is among the most common—and arguably the most important—mental disorders experienced while near the end of life due to its significant impact on quality of life, behavior, and communication. It often develops in individuals who already have dementia. Delirium undermines meaningful interaction with family, so treasure the moments when your loved one is lucid, alert, and interacting. Some choose to document these treasured interactions in a notebook or journal for others to enjoy.

Delirium is a secondary mental disorder and part of the disease process characterized by confusion, reduced awareness, memory problems, sleep disturbances, inattention, aggression, combativeness, and perceptual disturbances (hallucinations). It is highly prevalent among individuals dying of cancer during their final weeks of life, with up to 90 percent experiencing it.[47,48] It is important that visits by loved ones who preceded the dying individual in death (i.e., dead family members) not be mistaken for delirium. Visits from those on the other side of the veil can help guide your loved one through the process of passing into the next life. These encounters are comforting and don't require medical intervention.

Delirium is categorized (subtyped) based on whether the patient is restless (agitated or hyperactive delirium) or lethargic (quiet or hypoactive delirium). If a person experiences elements of both hyperactive and hypoactive delirium it is considered mixed delirium. Hypoactive or mixed delirium is the most common. Delirium is intimately connected with pain. Pain can worsen delirium symptoms, and mental exertion to cope with pain can cause diminished mental capacity.

Typical causes of delirium include side effects of treatment (chemotherapy drugs, steroids, antiemetics, opioids, withdrawal of opioids or benzodiazepines, antivirals, anticholinergics, and brain radiotherapy), uncontrolled pain, fecal impaction, full bladder, urinary tract infection, failure of vital organs, blood sugar imbalance, nutritional deficiencies (thiamine, folate, B12), or dehydration. Identifying a cause improves the management of delirium.

Some practical strategies to reduce delirium include the following:

- Make sure eyeglasses and hearing aides are available to reduce misinterpretations.
- Keep your loved one in a familiar environment (home) whenever possible. If not possible, place familiar objects near him or her.
- Minimize medical testing and interventions that are not absolutely necessary.
- Limit the number of visitors at one time.
- Reduce noxious stimuli and distressing stimuli (excessive heat or cold, bright lights).

Memory function, cognitive abilities, sensory perception, and overall well-being can be aided with essential oils. Scientists have observed that essential oils rich in 1,8-cineole (rosemary, Spanish sage) improve memory function, cognitive performance, and attention by altering the amount of acetylcholine available to the brain and protecting neurons against damage.[49] Most of this research has surrounded the oral administration (about 1.5 drops) of Spanish sage (*Salvia lavandulifolia*) and sage (*Salvia officinalis*) essential oil. However, since oral administration in a capsule may be difficult and increases the risk of interaction with medications, inhalation may be a better approach.

Fortunately, scientists have demonstrated that 1,8-cineole triggers neurochemical pathways involved in memory function and this can be achieved through inhalation of rosemary.[50,51] Rosemary also improves focus, alertness, and clarity and enhances mood when inhaled.[52] Additional beneficial essential oils include lavender and ylang ylang, which both influence dopamine levels and can produce a general calming effect. To manage delirium, add three drops of rosemary essential oil to a cotton ball and have your loved one inhale from this for five minutes. Another option is to add two drops of rosemary and one drop each of lavender and ylang ylang to the cotton ball. Refresh the cotton ball at least twice daily and allow your loved one to inhale as needed or desired. Alternately, diffuse rosemary (possibly with lavender and ylang ylang) essential oil for thirty minutes three to four times daily. Rosemary essential oil may allow you to have more cherished moments free from delirium due to its noteworthy effects on the brain.

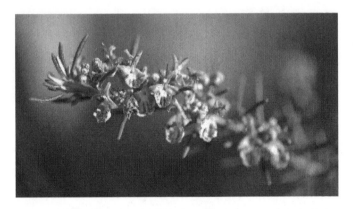

Loss of Mental Capacity

The ability to understand and make decisions for oneself relates to mental capacity. It involves the ability to comprehend, retain, weigh, and communicate information related to a particular decision. You should be prepared for the possibility that your loved one will lose his or her mental capacity. Major financial, social, and medical treatment decisions should be made early after the diagnosis of terminal illness whenever possible.

Outside of early decisions, you can use the rosemary essential oil method above to support cognitive well-being and mental capacity for as long as possible.

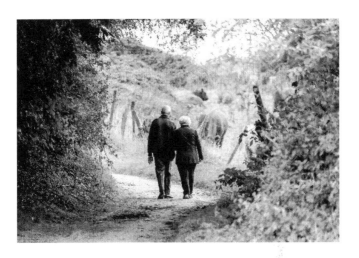

SPIRITUAL CHALLENGES

The spiritual challenges of dying are particularly difficult to navigate because of the lack of consensus on what spirituality means, who should address spiritual needs, and what appropriate actions to take. Despite this lack of clarity, the need to address spiritual care remains important. Indeed, many professionals consider spiritual care a basic tenet of end-of-life care.

Your loved one may be very introspective after a terminal diagnosis as he or she weighs his or her current relationship with God. Your loved one may be assessing the meaning and purpose of life—specifically his or her personal life. Or your loved one could be evaluating connections with beloved individuals and friends. All of this can lead to spiritual suffering as the impending death is anticipated and prepared for.

Loved ones of the person dying often feel similar emotions. They may be concerned about what happens to their loved one in the next life. Or they could be struggling with the thoughts of losing a deep spiritual connection. This is especially true for parent-child relationships. The need to address the spiritual needs of all involved cannot be overstated.

Some practical strategies to promote spiritual comfort include the following:

- Talk to a trusted spiritual leader (minister, priest, rabbi, cleric, or bishop).
- Speak with friends and family to resolve unsettled issues.
- A visit with a social worker or therapist.
- Share memories of good times and important past events.
- Prayer.
- Read religious texts.
- Listen to religious music.
- Tell your loved one the importance of your relationship and what it means to you, especially how he or she has positively influenced the course of your life.

Aromatic essences have been used for spiritual purposes for as long as recorded history. Ancient Egyptians burned incense as an offering to their gods. The Bible contains references to burning incense as part of sacred ceremonies, and the precious aromatic spices of frankincense and myrrh were given as gifts to the Christ child by wise men. Similarly, other cultures—Romans, Greeks, Indians, Chinese, and Persians—used aromatic essences for religious and spiritual purposes.

Today is no different. Some individuals still rely on essential oils to open the mind, enhance spiritual connections, and invite inspiration. This practice may also focus the mind to remove obstacles (i.e., emotional disturbances) that hinder reaching your full potential. While certainly not necessary to enhance spirituality or connect with God, the following essential oils are commonly inhaled or applied topically to the crown of the head to promote spirituality:

- *Cleansing and purification.* Angelica, anise, balsam fir, cedarwood, cypress, eucalyptus, juniper, lemon, lemon tea tree, myrrh, opoponax, peppermint, sage, spearmint, and white sage.
- *Grounding and inner focus.* Balsam fir, cedarwood, cinnamon, cypress, gurjun

balsam, mastic, palo santo, patchouli, pine, sandalwood, spruce, and vetiver.

- *Enlightenment and meditation.* Agarwood, balsam fir, cypress, elemi, frankincense, guaiacwood, guggul, myrrh, palo santo, sandalwood, spikenard, and Western red cedar.

- *Reconnection to a sense of spirituality.* Cassia, cinnamon, balsam fir, frankincense, ginger, lavender, myrtle, pine, sandalwood, and spruce (black).

HELPFUL ESSENTIAL OIL TIPS

- **Keep essential oils away from eyes**. If essential oils do get into the eyes by mistake, add a vegetable oil to the eye and pat the eye dry with a clean paper towel. Continue this process until relief is achieved. Do not use water as this will make the situation worse.

- **If skin irritation occurs add more carrier oil.** Some essential oils may irritate the skin of certain individuals. This can be alleviated by adding more carrier oil to the site of application until irritation subsides.

- **Avoid direct sunlight or UV rays for up to 12 hours after the topical use of certain oils.** Lemon (cold-pressed, CP), bergamot (CP), lime (CP), tangerine (CP), mandarin (CP), angelica, and cumin are essential oils mentioned in this text that may contain constituents (furano-coumarins) that increase sensitivity to UV rays and the risk of skin reactions. Steam-distilled citrus oils do not carry the same warning.

Transitional Stage

When confronted with the impending death of a loved one, many of us wonder when exactly death will occur. This is important to ensure adequate time for loved ones to say goodbye whenever possible. Keeping a vigil is a common practice so that loved ones can be at the bedside as their loved one passes. The question of how much time is left is difficult to answer, but there are signs and indications that can be used as a guide.

Caregivers should be aware of the transitional stage of dying, a stage that usually signifies that death is quickly approaching. A person's last weeks or months may include plateaus or a slow decline in functions that is your loved one's attempt at compensating for adjustments in psychophysiological performance. Attention to certain signs may help you better prepare for the actual time of death.

Two phases precede the actual time of death: the preactive phase of dying and the active stage of dying. The preactive stage typically lasts one to two weeks. On average, the active stage is much shorter, lasting about three days.

Signs and symptoms of the preactive stage of dying

- Increased sleeping or lethargy
- Increased restlessness and agitation
- Social withdrawal
- Increased swelling (extremities or entire body)
- Pauses in breathing (apnea) while awake or while sleeping
- Reports of seeing people who preceded your loved one in death
- Wounds or infections that won't heal
- Decreased intake of food or liquids
- Your loved one states he or she is dying

Signs and symptoms of the active stage of dying

- Great effort or inability to awaken your loved one

- Increased terminal secretions; death rattle
- Long periods of pauses in breathing, very rapid breathing, or cyclic changes in breathing
- Severe agitation
- Hallucinations or behavior not normal for your loved one
- Urinary or bowel incontinence; marked decrease in urine output or dark urine
- Inability to swallow fluids
- Dramatic drops in blood pressure (20+ point drop); blood pressure below 70/50
- Cold extremities (hands, feet, arms, legs)
- Numbness in the legs or feet
- Skin mottling (bluish or purple coloring of the extremities), which may begin at the toes and fingers and gradually work toward the center of the body
- Rigid or unchanging body position
- Jaw drop (not straight and may drop toward the side his or her head is leaning)

Conclusion

We will all face the death of a loved one at some point during our lifetimes. We may even be contemplating our own destiny with death. Early preparation and having a group of essential oils prepared beforehand can lead to improved overall care of your loved one. Learning the techniques and strategies now will reduce stress when you receive the opportunity to provide compassionate care for your loved one. Being prepared may also ease your loved one's suffering and help him or her transition more successfully to the next life. Essential oils can make this special time a cherished memory for both the one nearing the end of life and those providing compassionate care.

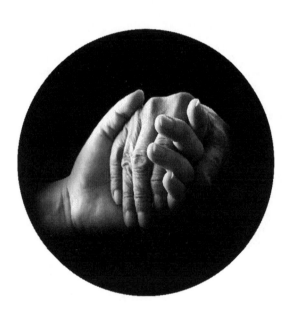

REFERENCES

[1] Gatchel RJ. Comorbidity of chronic pain and mental health disorders: The biopsychosocial perspective. *Am Psychol.* 2004 Nov;59(8):795-805.

[2] Lumley MA, Cohen JL, Borszcz GS, et al. Pain and Emotion: A Biopsychosocial Review of Recent Research. *J Clin Psychol.* 2011 Sep;67(9):942–968.

[3] Bushnell MC, Ceko M, Low LA. Cognitive and emotional control of pain and its disruption in chronic pain. *Nat Rev Neurosci.* 2013 Jul; 14(7): 502–511.

[4] McCann RM, Hall WJ, Groth-Juncker A. Comfort care for terminally ill patients. The appropriate use of nutrition and hydration. *JAMA.* 1994;272:1263–6.

[5] Torelli GF, Campos AC, Meguid MM. Use of TPN in terminally ill cancer patients. *Nutrition.* 1999;15:665–7.

[6] Cohn SH, Vartsky D, Vaswani AN, et al. Changes in body composition of cancer patients following combined nutritional support. *Nutr Cancer.* 1982;4(2):107-19.

[7] Fine RL. Ethical issues in artificial nutrition and hydration. *Nutr Clin Pract.* 2006;21(2):118-125.

[8] Klein S, Koretz RL. Nutrition support in patients with cancer: What do the data really show? *Nutr Clin Pract.* 1994;9(3):91-100.

[9] Finucane TE, Christmas C, Travis K. Tube feeding in patients with advanced dementia: A review of the evidence. *JAMA.* 1999;282(14):1365-1370.

[10] Mitchell SL, Kiely DK, Lipsitz LA. Does artificial enteral nutrition prolong the survival of institutionalized elders with chewing and swallowing problems? *J Gerontol.* 1998;53(3):M207-M213.

[11] Ellershaw JE, Sutcliffe JM, Saunders M. Dehydration and the dying patient. *J Pain Symptom Manage.* 1995;10(3):192-197.

[12] McCann RM, Hall WJ, Groth-Junker A. Comfort care for terminally ill patients. The appropriate use of nutrition and hydration. *JAMA.* 1994;272(16):1253-1266.

[13] Shen J, Niijima A, Tanida M, et al. Olfactory stimulation with scent of lavender oil affects autonomic nerves, lipolysis and appetite in rats. *Neurosci Lett.* 2005 Jul 22-29;383(1-2):188-93.

[14] Ogawa K, Ito M. Appetite-Enhancing Effects of Curry Oil. *Biol Pharm Bull.* 2016;39(9):1559-63.

[15] Ogawa K, Ito M, et al. Appetite-enhancing Effects of trans-Cinnamaldehyde, Benzylacetone and 1-Phenyl-2-butanone by Inhalation. *Planta Med.* 2016 Jan;82(1-2):84-8. d

[16] Vazquez JA, Zawawi AA. Efficacy of alcohol-based and alcohol-free melaleuca oral solution for the treatment of fluconazole-refractory oropharyngeal candidiasis in patients with AIDS. *HIV Clin Trials.* 2002 Sep-Oct;3(5):379-85.

[17] Kang HY, Na SS, Kim YK. Effects of Oral Care with Essential Oil on Improvement in Oral Health Status of Hospice Patients. *J Korean Acad Nurs.* 2010;40(4):473-481.

[18] Ebihara T, Ebihara S, Maruyama M, et al. A randomized trial of olfactory stimulation using black pepper oil in older people with swallowing dysfunction. *J Am Geriatr Soc.* 2006 Sep;54(9):1401-06.

[19] Wee B, Hillier R. Interventions for noisy breathing in patients near death (Review). *Cochrane Database Systematic Reviews.* 2010;2:1-17

[20] Wildiers H, Dhaenekint C, Demeulenaere P, et al. Atropine, Hyoscine Butylbromide, or Scopolamine Are Equally Effective for the Treatment of Death Rattle in Terminal Care' Journal of Pain and Symptom Management. 2009;38(1):124-33.

[21] Johnson SA. Medicinal Essential Oils: The Science and Practice of Evidence-Based Essential Oil Therapy. 2017 Aug. Scott A Johnson Professional Writing Services, LLC: Orem, Utah.

[22] Kohara H, Miyauchi T, Suehiro Y, et al. Combined Modality Treatment of Aromatherapy, Footsoak, and Reflexology Relieves Fatigue in Patients with Cancer. *J Palliative Med.* 2004 Dec;7(6):791-6.

[23] Varney E, Buckle J. Effect of inhaled essential oils on mental exhaustion and moderate burnout: a small pilot study. *J Altern Complement Med.* 2013;19(1):69-71.

[24] Glare P, Miller J, Nikolova T, et al. Treating nausea and vomiting in palliative care: a review. *Clin Interv Aging.* 2011;6:243-59.

[25] Rousseau P. Nonpain symptom management in the dying patient. *Hospital Physician.* 2002:51-56.

[26] Richards A. Hands on help. *N Times.* 1998;94:69–73

[27] Kim MA, Sakong JK, Kim EJ, et al. [Effect of aromatherapy massage for the relief of constipation in the elderly]. *Taehan Kanho Hakhoe Chi.* 2005 Feb;35(1):56-64.

[28] Hugel H, Ellershaw JE, Cook L, et al. The prevalence, key causes and management of insomnia in palliative care patients. *J Pain Symptom Manage.* 2004;27(4):316.

[29] Mercadante S, Aielli F, Adile C, et al. Sleep Disturbances in Patients With Advanced Cancer in Different Palliative Care Settings. *J Pain Symptom Manage.* 2015 Dec;50(6):786-92.

[30] Lytle J, Mwatha C, Davis KK. Effect of lavender aromatherapy on vital signs and perceived quality of sleep in the intermediate care unit: a pilot study. *Am J Crit Care.* 2014 Jan;23(1):24-29.

[31] Johannessen B. Nurses experience of aromatherapy use with dementia patients experiencing disturbed sleep patterns. An action research project. *Complement Ther Clin Pract.* 2013 Nov;19(4):209-13.

[32] Goel N, Kim H, Lao RP. An olfactory stimulus modifies sleep in young men and women. *Chronobiol Int.* 2005;22(5):889-904.

[33] Lewith GT, Godfrey AD, Prescott P. A single-blinded, randomized pilot study evaluating the aroma of Lavandula angustifolia as a treatment for mild insomnia. *J Altern Complement Med.* 2005 Aug;11(4):631-17.

[34] Park H, Chun Y, Kwak S. The Effects of Aroma Hand Massage on Fatigue and Sleeping among Hospice Patients. *Open J Nursing.* 2016;6:515-23.

[35] Maignana Kumar R, Rukmani A, Saradha S, et al. Evaluation of antiepileptic activity of vetiveria zizanioides oil in mice. *Int J Pharm Sci Rev Res.* 2014 Mar-Apr;25(2):248-51.

[36] de Sousaa DP, Nóbregab FF, de Morais LC, et al. Evaluation of the Anticonvulsant Activity of Terpinen-4-ol. *Z Naturforsch C*. 2009 Jan-Feb;64(1-2):1-5.

[37] Nirwane AM, Gupta PV, Shet JH, et al. Anxiolytic and nootropic activity of Vetiveria zizanioides roots in mice. *J Ayurveda Integr Med*. 2015 Jul-Sep; 6(3):158-64.

[38] Rajasekhar CH, Kokila BN, Rajesh B. Potential effect of Vetiveria Zizanioides root extract and essential oil on phenobarbital induced sedation-hypnosis in Swiss albino mice. *Int J Exp Pharmacol*. 2014;4:89–93.

[39] Arzi A, Sela L, Green A, et al. The influence of odorants on respiratory patterns in sleep. *Chem Senses*. 2010 Jan;35(1):31-40.

[40] Dyer J, Cleary L, McNeill S, et al. The use of aromasticks to help with sleep problems: A patient experience survey. *Complement Ther Clin Pract*. 2016 Feb;22:51-8.

[41] Cleary JF, Carbone PP. Palliative medicine in the elderly. *Cancer*. 1997 Oct 1; 80(7):1335-47.

[42] Parker Oliver D, Washington K, Smith J, et al. The Prevalence and Risks for Depression and Anxiety in Hospice Caregivers. *J Palliat Med*. 2017 Apr;20(4):366-371.

[43] Wilkinson S. Aromatherapy and massage in palliative care. *Int J Palliat Nurs*. 1995 Jan 2;1(1):21-30.

[44] Wilkinson S, Aldridge J, Salmon I, et al. An evaluation of aromatherapy massage in palliative care. *Palliat Med*. 1999 Sep;13(5):409-17.

[45] Chang SY. Effects of Aroma Hand Massage on Pain, State Anxiety and Depression in Hospice Patients with Terminal Cancer. *J Korean Acad Nurs*. 2008 Aug;38(4):493-502.

[46] Louis M, Kowalski SD. Use of aromatherapy with hospice patients to decrease pain, anxiety, and depression and to promote an increased sense of well-being. *Am J Hosp Palliat Care*. 2002 Nov-Dec;19(6):381-6.

[47] Kang JH, Shin SH, Bruera E. Comprehensive Approaches to Managing Delirium in Patients with Advanced Cancer. *Cancer Treat Rev*. 2013 Feb;39(1):10.

[48] Fang CK, Chen HW, Liu SI, et al. Prevalence, Detection and Treatment of Delirium in Terminal Cancer Inpatients: A Prospective Survey. *Japanese J Clin Oncology.* 2008 Jan;38(1):53-63.

[49] Johnson SA. Medicinal Essential Oils: The Science and Practice of Evidence-Based Essential Oil Therapy. 2017 Aug. Scott A Johnson Professional Writing Services, LLC: Orem, Utah.

[50] Moss M, Cook J, Wesnes K, et al. Aromas of rosemary and lavender essential oils differentially affect cognition and mood in healthy adults. *Int J Neurosci.* 2003 Jan;113(1):15-38.

[51] Moss M, Oliver L. Plasma 1,8-cineole correlates with cognitive performance following exposure to rosemary essential oil aroma. *Ther Adv Psychopharmacol.* 2012 Jun;2(3):103-13.

[52] Johnson SA. Medicinal Essential Oils: The Science and Practice of Evidence-Based Essential Oil Therapy. 2017 Aug. Scott A Johnson Professional Writing Services, LLC: Orem, Utah.

Made in the USA
Columbia, SC
16 May 2022

60486895R00043